Intermittent Fasting:
A Beginners Guide

Jason Legend

ISBN: 9781691619634

DEDICATION

This book is dedicated to everyone who's ever worked out with me, and pushed me to become better.

CONTENTS

Chapter 1

Introduction

Intermittent fasting is a rapidly growing popular trend to weight loss, fitness, and health in the whole world. Intermittent fasting is changing the eating patterns or schedules to obtain good health and to lose weight. It does not restrict what to eat or not, but it makes a proper schedule of when to eat. Intermittent fasting is concerned with eating periods instead of what to eat. [1] It is a combination of the appropriate timing of when to eat and when to fast. Usually, people do tend to fast every day; for example, they do not eat when they are sleeping or busy in some work. However, intermittent fasting is maintaining such a proper schedule to allocate the eating and fasting periods per day, week, or month. So for example, you can skip breakfast at a regular time (when you wake up), and you wait until eating your first food at noon and your last meal at 8 pm. That means 16 hours fasting (not eating) each day, which restricts the hours for eating at 8-hour intervals. Doing that is one of the most popular intermittent fasting methods, which is also known as the 16/8 method; since you're fasting for 16 hours a day, and eating for 8. [1] [2]

So, intermittent fasting is time-restricted eating with proper and strict timing control to get its benefits. Typically, people start eating as they wake up and stop eating when they go to bed. They do not have any proper schedule of when to eat and when not to eat. [11] People do not eat continuously, but most people typically eat three times a day: breakfast, lunch, and dinner. Even though most people eat those three meals, with snacks in between and even sometimes after dinner, they don't have any hard cut-off time to starting and stopping eating. Time-restricted eating is based on a schedule, like eating for 8 hours and fasting for 16 hours. So, intermittent fasting is time-restricted eating with proper and strict timing control to get its benefits. [2]

It does not mean that intermittent fasting results in losing energy and feeling bad. However, it can improve your mental state, with more energy levels. It may cause some ill-feelings, like hunger in beginning periods as people are not used to fasting. Intermittent fasting typically only restricts eating rather than drinking so that people can drink non-caloric beverages. While some of the intermittent fasting methods also allow a small number of low-calorie foods to be eaten even during fasting as well.

Intermittent fasting is more effective than limiting yourself to certain types of foods. However, its timing is essential to obtain the required results. Intermittent fasting results typically in 3–8% weight loss in 3 – 24 weeks. It also can improve your metabolism.

Chapter 2

Brief History of Intermittent Fasting

Fasting has a long back history from ancient times as people were fasting from thousands of years ago. Although it was due to some acute shortage of foods, it also became part of peoples' lives. It was used for health, weight loss, fitness, and a religious basis as well. World-famous religions, such as Christianity, Islam, and Buddhism, have put mandatory fasting for their followers. [2]

On the other hand, fasting is natural as our body has the capability for extended non-eating periods like fasting. In ancient times, people were eating foods for survival rather than taste and enjoyment, like today. They were getting food from hunting, fishing, and gathering, so they had to fast until they could find their next meal.

There were no breakfast, lunch, and dinner routines. They ate as they found anything to eat; otherwise, they had to fast, which may extend to days and weeks. Therefore, people tried to live alongside lakes, rivers, mountains, and forest areas where they could get their foods. [5]

Muslims fast during the holy month of Ramadan for almost 30 days according to their lunar months which duration may differ according to season and day lengths.

Muslim fasting may extend up to 14-15 hours. Roman Catholics and Eastern Orthodoxy intermittently fast for 40 days during the Lent period. In religious practices, fasting is taken as a holiness sign along with health benefits. It means that world religions have put mandatory fasting for their followers. Religions institutions were aware of its benefits and importance from the beginning of the world. [6]

Fasting also remained part of political and social protest in the world. History is full of hunger strikes by different leaders for their rights. Mahatma Gandhi is one of them, as he fasted many times, including a 21-day hunger strike. In 1928, Dr. Herbert Shelton opened "Dr. Shelton's Health School in Texas and claimed to help about 40 thousand patients' disease recovery with a water fast. In 1920, the Nature Cure approach adopted fasting as a popular treatment in the United Kingdom. The first Nature Cure clinic, which opened in

Edinburgh, offers intermittent fasting as a treatment practice. Fasting was recommended for high blood pressure, heart diseases, headaches, allergies, digestive issues, and obesity. [6]

Although intermittent fasting is a long-lasting concept among humans, it was popularized explicitly as intermittent fasting by BBC journalist Dr. Michael Mosley's TV documentary "Eat, Fast, Live Longer", and the book "The Fast Diet" in 2012. Subsequently, "The 5:2 Diet" book of journalist Kate Harrison, and Dr. Jason Fung's book "The Obesity Code" popularized it. [13]

Chapter 3

How Intermittent Fasting Works

To understand how intermittent fasting works, we need to understand the difference between a fasted state and a fed state of our body. Typically, our body remains in a fed state when we are eating, and our body is digesting/absorbing foods. A fed state starts as we start eating, and lasts for 3–5 hours when our body digests and absorbs the food. It is difficult for our body to burn fat during a fed state as insulin levels are high. After absorption of food when our body is free from processing the meal, the body enters into a fasted state. In the fasted state, fat burning is more natural, as insulin levels are much lower where our body becomes enabled to burn excessive fats. So, intermittent fasting puts our body in a fat-burning state that is rarely achievable in regular eating habits.

As you start fasting, many things start happening on cellular and molecular levels in your body. The human body starts adjusting hormone levels to access body fats. Cells digest more and remove dysfunctional old proteins from cells. Intermittent fasting stimulates cells to initiate vital repair processes and change expressions of genes in the human body. Gene expressions change genes' longevity and help to protect from diseases. [1]

Intermittent fasting allows human

bodies to thrive during fasting. It reduces blood sugar and insulin levels in human bodies and drastically increases growth hormones. Intermittent fasting is the most natural and most effective process to burn fats and restrains calories during weight loss.

Intermittent fasting improves the balance of fat-burning hormones, making it that much more helpful to manage weight. Insulin hormones are involved in body fat metabolism as it directs the human body to store fat and stop breaking fat down. Taking higher levels of insulin makes it much more difficult to lose weight for the human body. Observing higher levels of insulin can lead to some severe diseases like cancer, obesity, heart disease, and type 2 diabetes. Intermittent fasting restricts higher calorie consumption and lowers insulin levels that save from diseases and excessive storage of insulin and metabolism. Intermittent fasting typically reduces insulin levels 20–30% in the human body. [3]

Chapter 4

Types of Intermittent Fasting

Intermittent fasting is very simple, as it is choosing some specific time window to eat all of your required calories each day. If someone takes his/her first meal at 7 am and keeps eating around 10 pm or else near about it, it means they are eating for approximately 15 hours a day. Now, he/she has to reduce and restrict himself/herself for some 8–9 hours daily during intermittent fasting. It will limit one or more meals or some snacks from routine eating.

Intermittent fasting is not a forced timing or strict schedule that everyone has to act or comply with set rules. It is a simple, easy, and adjustable eating pattern, which allows people to set their own schedule as per their feasibility and convenience. It can be adopted as a single method or way of intermittent fasting, or to take a mixture of some methods. It depends upon the requirement and the will of the person to adopt their suitable approach for intermittent fasting. Anyone can make his own intermittent fasting schedule or copy any one of the set methods.

Numbers of intermittent fasting methods, ways, and types have been evolved during the time-periods from ancient times to the present era. Numerous health and fitness experts have worked on intermittent fasting methods, schedules, and plans. They have evolved some excellent intermittent fasting methods which are beneficial for most people. They have set methods that can be adopted by almost anyone, without any difficulty. Some of the most popular types of intermittent fasting are: [2]

The 16/8

The 16/8 method is also known as the Leangains protocol. Fitness expert Martin Berkhan introduced this. Intermittent fasting in this method is simple. It typically requires that you do not eat after dinner, and also skip the typical breakfast. If someone feels that it is too hard to skip breakfast, he can drink non-caloric beverages and water even during fasting times.

It consists of fasting for 16 hours a day. Mostly, people adopt eating between noon and 8 pm. As previously stated, it can be achieved by eating your first meal at noon and eating your second meal at 8 pm. Now there would be 16 hours gap between second to first meal and 8 hours gap between the first to the second meal. That's why we call it the 16/8 method of intermittent fasting. It can be scheduled from 1 – 9 pm, eating your first meal at 1 pm and your second meal at 9 pm. Alternatively, these timing can be changed as per your convenience, but there should be 8 hours gap between first and second meal and 16 hours gap between second and first meal. [1] [7]

Mostly, people like to adopt 16/8 intermittent fasting as their preferred method, as it is practical and straightforward. Some of the top fitness experts and intermittent fasting lovers have adopted this method and reviewed it to be the best one among all of the intermittent fasting methods.

Eat-Stop-Eat

Eat-Stop-Eat intermittent fasting method is 24 hours of fasting, or whole day fasting, once or twice per week. Brad Pilon, a fitness expert, introduced this method. It is not easy for everyone, though. It can be difficult to not eat for 24 hours. [7]

It is the best way to get intermittent fasting done once or twice in a week or even a month. It is also known as occasional fasting or weekly fasting. This method is typically most comfortable to do by not eating from dinner to the next dinner once or twice a week. For example, do not eat anything from Monday's dinner to Tuesday's dinner. It can also be adopted, possibly easier, by not eating from breakfast to breakfast. If you eat breakfast on Monday morning, it might be easy not to eat all day, go to sleep, and wake up to breakfast on Tuesday. This way you're sleeping through your hungriest part.

It can also be adopted, of course, as

fasting from lunch to lunch as long as you are going 24 hours without eating. As previously stated, this can be a convenient way for someone who wants to intermittent fast periodically, but not every day.

You can prepare some other schedules or plans as you see fit. It depends on your capacity to choose which day should be for fasting and which day to eat. Some people prefer holidays for fasting while others prefer eating out and enjoying holidays. Similarly, some people prefer fasting when they are at home while others prefer fasting when they are in the office. So, it depends on people's will, availability, and convenience.

5: 2 Diet

The 5:2 diet practices healthy eating for five days and 500-600 calories restriction on two days of the week. [1] This diet is also popular as a fast diet. British journalist Dr. Michael Mosley introduced the method. Women are recommended to eat 500 calories, while men are advised to eat 600 calories during the fasting period. However, it could be modified to be 250 and 300 calories for women and men, respectively.

It is eating only about 500-600 calories for two days a week. These two days can be chosen according to one's convenience. However, these two days should be non-consecutive days of a week. For example, it can be Monday and Wednesday, Monday and Thursday, Monday and Friday, Tuesday and Friday, Tuesday and Saturday, Wednesday and Friday, Wednesday and Sunday or any else combination as per your convenience. [15]

Alternative Days

This method involves eating one day and not eating on the next consecutive day. It means eating and fasting kept on alternate days in weeks. For example, eating on Monday and fasting on Tuesday, eating on Wednesday and fasting on Thursday, eating on Friday and fasting on Saturday. It can be changed from day to day selection as appropriate for you.

Although similar to the Eat-Stop-Eat method, this method is adopted for more extended fasting periods throughout the week.

The Warrior Diet

The warrior diet method consists of fasting during the day and eating a good quantity meal during the night for dinner. A fitness expert Ori Hofmekler introduced this method. In this method, small amounts of raw fruits and vegetables are eaten during the day while a big healthy meal is eaten at night. [15]

Spontaneous Meal Skipping

This is a choice-based method or way of intermittent fasting. In this way, people have to skip eating or keep on fasting when convenient for them. Spontaneous meal skipping is a to intermittent fast, without having a structured schedule. Someone eats and fasts as per his feasibility or when not feeling hungry. Most people do this in one way or another in their everyday life without even realizing it.

The trick is to make your meals you do eat, be healthy. [15]

Chapter 5

Benefits of Intermittent Fasting

Intermittent fasting has many benefits for individual health and fitness, but it also keeps the society and overall environmental health. It not only maintains our health and fitness, but it also can help prevent many severe diseases as well. Some of the essential benefits are elaborated here.

Weight loss

Weight loss is one of the greater benefits of intermittent fasting, as obesity has become a serious disease that invites other diseases. Intermittent fasting is arguably the most effective way to weight loss vs. any other diet and medicines. Some research studies have claimed 5% weight loss during 2 – 4 weeks just due to 7 – 12 hours of intermittent fasting. However, it all depends on how many calories you eat during the day and how healthy the food is. Intermittent fasting helps to burn fats to help weight loss. Similarly, intermittent fasting controls insulin to help in fat burning for better health and weight loss. Intermittent fasting reduces calorie consumption, resulting in weight loss because controlled and restricted eating during fasting periods consumes fewer calories, which helps lose weight. [1] [14]

Change in hormone level during fasting also help to weight loss. People have reportedly lost 4–7 % of their waist circumference, especially belly fat, during intermittent fasting.[4]

Heart Health

Intermittent fasting is beneficial for heart health too. Human blood carries cholesterol. While low-density lipoprotein (LDL) cholesterol is bad for heart health, high-density lipoprotein (HDL) is good for heart health. HDL decreases heart disease risks, while LDL increases heart disease risk. Intermittent fasting has been shown to lower bad LDL, which ultimately lowers the risk of heart diseases. [14]

Blood Sugar

Sugar, or glucose, is essential for human health, but its excessive quantity in human blood may cause diabetes and damage body parts leading toward severe diseases. Intermittent fasting remains helpful in controlling sugar levels in the blood to protect from diseases. [14]

Consistency and Patience

Intermittent fasting brings consistency in eating. Whatever you have to eat and when you have to eat; you will eat it with proper consistency. You have to follow your schedule; otherwise, you will not be able to get all of the benefits of intermittent fasting. So, consistency is vital during intermittent fasting, and it makes a habit of consistent eating during your whole life. Similarly, intermittent fasting leads toward patience and will-power during fasting periods, as you have to keep will-power even when you're feeling hungry, contrary to your fasting times. [14]

Overall Health

Intermittent fasting improves health. It can be an effective and natural way for better health, rather than any medical treatment. Intermittent fasting reduces insulin resistance and lowers blood sugar that protects from type 2 diabetes and other diseases, and reduces inflammation markers to prevent other chronic diseases. [1] Intermittent fasting is good for brain health, as it proves helpful to increase the brain hormone BDNF and promotes the growth of new nerve cells. It expands life span with good health. Intermittent fasting reduces oxidative damage and inflammation in the human body. Oxidative stress is one of the leading causes of aging and other chronic diseases. [14]

Chapter 6

Disadvantages and Precautions for Intermittent Fasting

Although intermittent fasting is suitable for most people, there are some precautions to avoid any mishap or risk to your health. Intermittent fasting can be dangerous or less effective in some cases, as it is not for everyone in every condition. The main problems from intermittent fasting can be hunger, loss of energy, health, and overall unpleasantness. It makes people miserable at work during fasting and low down their efficiency and proficiency. It may hurt them with weakness and laziness during the routine daily life. Depending on the method you're using, these "side effects" eventually go away, or dissipate. If someone has an eating disorder or is underweight, he should also consult with a doctor before trying intermittent fasting.[1]

Hunger is one of the main side effects of intermittent fasting, but it should be up to a reasonable control level. If someone tries intermittent fasting and cannot bear the hunger burden, he should reconsider it before adopting to intermittent fasting, or try a different method. Gradually, fasting habits should be chosen so your body should be able to adapt to these practices. If someone has any medical treatment or unique medical history, he should consult with a specialist or doctor. Intermittent fasting is not a cure for every panic, disease, and health issue. There is dire need to consult with a doctor before going on an intermittent fasting schedule, especially in the following cases. [1]

a. Low blood pressure.

b. Blood sugar regulation problems.

c. Diabetes

d. Taking medications

e. Eating disorder

f. Underweight

g. A woman trying to conceive

h. A woman has a history of amenorrhea

i. If a woman is pregnant

j. If a woman is breastfeeding

References

1. Kris Gunnars, Intermittent Fasting 101 — The Ultimate Beginner's Guide.
https://www.healthline.com/nutrition/intermittent-fasting-guide, Jul 25, 2018.

2. Kris Gunnars, What Is Intermittent Fasting? Explained in Human Terms.
https://www.healthline.com/nutrition/what-is-intermittent-fasting, Jun 4, 2017.

3. Helen West, Does Intermittent Fasting Boost Your Metabolism?
https://www.healthline.com/nutrition/intermittent-fasting-metabolism#section6, Nov 20, 2016

4. Kris Gunnars, How Intermittent Fasting Can Help You Lose Weight.
https://www.healthline.com/nutrition/intermittent-fasting-and-weight-loss#section6, Jun 4, 2017

5. Alexandra Pattillo, Is Intermittent Fasting "Natural"? History Experts Respond to the Controversy Leave our ancestors out of it.
https://www.inverse.com/article/57835-intermittent-fasting-evolution, Jul 26, 2019

6. Cherrill Hicks. Why fasting is now back in fashion.

https://www.telegraph.co.uk/lifestyle/11524808/The-history-of-fasting.html, Apr 13, 2015

7. Steve Kamb, Intermittent Fasting: Beginner's Guide & Printable Calendar. Should You Skip Breakfast, https://www.nerdfitness.com/blog/a-beginners-guide-to-intermittent-fasting/, Jul 29, 2019

8. Kris Gunnars, 11 Myths about Fasting and Meal Frequency, https://www.healthline.com/nutrition/11-myths-fasting-and-meal-frequency, Jul 22, 2019

9. Kris Gunnars, How Many Calories Should You Eat Per Day to Lose Weight?, https://www.healthline.com/nutrition/how-many-calories-per-day#section4, Jul 6, 2018

10. Kris Gunnars, How to Lose Weight Fast: 3 Simple Steps, Based on Science. https://www.healthline.com/nutrition/how-to-lose-weight-as-fast-as-possible, Mar 14, 2018

11. Grant Tinsley, Time-Restricted Eating: A Beginner's Guide. https://www.healthline.com/nutrition/time-restricted-eating, Sep 17, 2017

12. Kris Gunnars, 26 Weight Loss Tips That Are Actually Evidence-Based,. https://www.healthline.com/nutrition/26-evidence-based-weight-loss-tips#section25, Aug 22, 2018

13. Monique Tello, Intermittent fasting: Surprising update.https://www.health.harvard.edu/blog/intermittent-fasting-surprising-updte-2018062914156, Jun 29, 2018

14. Kris Gunnars, 10 Evidence-Based Health Benefits of Intermittent Fasting. https://www.healthline.com/nutrition/10-health-benefits-of-intermittent-fasting, Aug 16, 2016

15. Kris Gunnars, 6 Popular Ways to Do Intermittent Fasting. https://www.healthline.com/nutrition/6-ways-to-do-intermittent-fasting, Jun 4, 2017

16. Ryan Raman, Water Fasting: Benefits and Dangers. https://www.healthline.com/nutrition/water-fasting, Oct 22, 2017